Healing with Essential Oils

35 Recipes for Different Illnesses

Table of Contents

Introduction

You keep your house clean, you keep your dishes clean, you wash your hands often, and you avoid people who are sick. Yet, in spite of all your hard work, it seems that you can't get away from the illness, and when it strikes, it hangs on.

You don't like the side effects that come with modern medicine, but you know you can't just lie around feeling terrible, either. You need something that will get you back on your feet and up and around again, without bringing you a lot of harmful side effects along with it.

That's where essential oils come in. Used for thousands of years because of their incredible healing properties, these oils are known for healing and promoting a healthy lifestyle.

With the right blends, you have everything you need to heal your aches and pains without any of the harmful side effects that come with modern medicine.

But how do you know which of these blends to use?

How do you know which oils work for the illness you are experiencing?

How do you know how to use the oils for the best health possible?

You are going to learn the answer to all these questions and more with this book, and you're going to find the blends that will get you up on your feet and out the door. This book holds the recipes you need to cure any illness, and it will give you what you need to stay healthy, even in the cold and flu season.

I am going to show you a variety of blends, and you can use them all for any illness you catch. Whether you use a diffuser or directly apply them to the affected area, you are going to find that these oils are the answer you have been waiting for.

So grab your oils and get blending.

You have a healthy life to live.

Chapter 1 – The Recipes

Cold Crasher

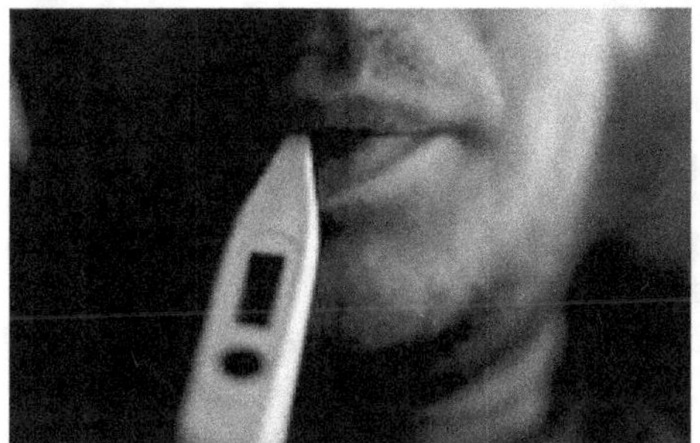

What you will need:

10 drops grapefruit oil

8 drops lime oil

Direct Application Directions:

Mix the blend well, and if you are going to apply it directly to your skin mix with 2 teaspoons sweet almond oil and spread over the affected area. You may also mix with the lotion of your choice – do not ingest the oils.

Repeat every couple hours, or as often as needed.

Diffuser Directions:

Fill your diffuser with water according to the directions on the packaging, then add a few drops of this blend, also according to the packaging. Plug in your

diffuser and place it where you will be able to sit or sleep nearby, and breathe in the mist.

Continue to mist as needed.

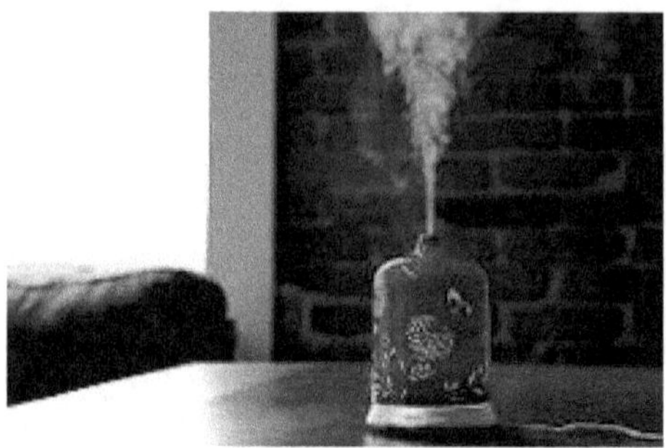

Sore Throat Soother
What you will need:

18 drops peppermint oil

12 drops lime oil

Direct Application Directions:

Mix the blend well, and if you are going to apply it directly to your skin mix with 2 teaspoons sweet almond oil and spread over the affected area. You may also mix with the lotion of your choice – do not ingest the oils.

Repeat every couple hours, or as often as needed.

Diffuser Directions:

Fill your diffuser with water according to the directions on the packaging, then add a few drops of this blend, also according to the packaging. Plug in your diffuser and place it where you will be able to sit or sleep nearby, and breathe in the mist.

Continue to mist as needed.

The Cure All
What you will need:

9 drops patchouli oil

9 drops tea tree oil

Direct Application Directions:

Mix the blend well, and if you are going to apply it directly to your skin mix with 2 teaspoons sweet almond oil and spread over the affected area. You may also mix with the lotion of your choice – do not ingest the oils.

Repeat every couple hours, or as often as needed.

Diffuser Directions:

Fill your diffuser with water according to the directions on the packaging, then add a few drops of this blend, also according to the packaging. Plug in your diffuser and place it where you will be able to sit or sleep nearby, and breathe in the mist.

Continue to mist as needed.

All Better
What you will need:

10 drops cedar oil

9 drops sandalwood oil

Direct Application Directions:

Mix the blend well, and if you are going to apply it directly to your skin mix with 2 teaspoons sweet almond oil and spread over the affected area. You may also mix with the lotion of your choice – do not ingest the oils.

Repeat every couple hours, or as often as needed.

Diffuser Directions:

Fill your diffuser with water according to the directions on the packaging, then add a few drops of this blend, also according to the packaging. Plug in your diffuser and place it where you will be able to sit or sleep nearby, and breathe in the mist.

Continue to mist as needed.

Easy Street

What you will need:

8 drops geranium oil

9 drops grapefruit oil

Direct Application Directions:

Mix the blend well, and if you are going to apply it directly to your skin mix with 2 teaspoons sweet almond oil and spread over the affected area. You may also mix with the lotion of your choice – do not ingest the oils.

Repeat every couple hours, or as often as needed.

Diffuser Directions:

Fill your diffuser with water according to the directions on the packaging, then add a few drops of this blend, also according to the packaging. Plug in your

diffuser and place it where you will be able to sit or sleep nearby, and breathe in the mist.

Continue to mist as needed.

24 Hour Blend
What you will need:

12 drops clove oil

9 drops clary sage oil

Direct Application Directions:

Mix the blend well, and if you are going to apply it directly to your skin mix with 2 teaspoons sweet almond oil and spread over the affected area. You may also mix with the lotion of your choice – do not ingest the oils.

Repeat every couple hours, or as often as needed.

Diffuser Directions:

Fill your diffuser with water according to the directions on the packaging, then add a few drops of this blend, also according to the packaging. Plug in your diffuser and place it where you will be able to sit or sleep nearby, and breathe in the mist.

Continue to mist as needed.

Warm and Cozy

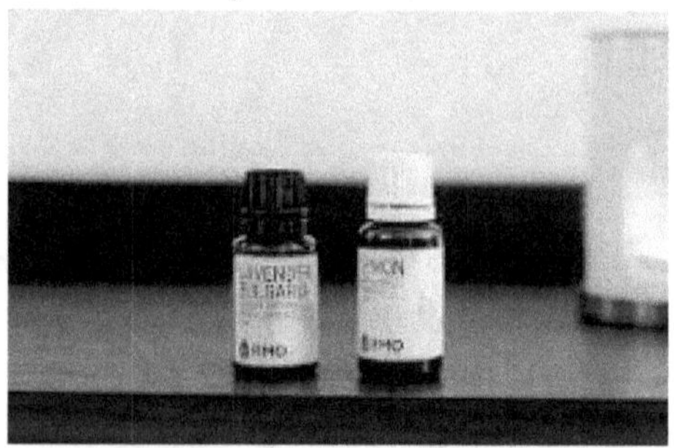

What you will need:

10 drops ginger oil

8 drops cinnamon oil

Direct Application Directions:

Mix the blend well, and if you are going to apply it directly to your skin mix with 2 teaspoons sweet almond oil and spread over the affected area. You may also mix with the lotion of your choice – do not ingest the oils.

Repeat every couple hours, or as often as needed.

Diffuser Directions:

Fill your diffuser with water according to the directions on the packaging, then add a few drops of this blend, also according to the packaging. Plug in your diffuser and place it where you will be able to sit or sleep nearby, and breathe in the mist.

Continue to mist as needed.

Like New
What you will need:

10 drops pine oil

8 drops winter green oil

Direct Application Directions:

Mix the blend well, and if you are going to apply it directly to your skin mix with 2 teaspoons sweet almond oil and spread over the affected area. You may also mix with the lotion of your choice – do not ingest the oils.

Repeat every couple hours, or as often as needed.

Diffuser Directions:

Fill your diffuser with water according to the directions on the packaging, then add a few drops of this blend, also according to the packaging. Plug in your diffuser and place it where you will be able to sit or sleep nearby, and breathe in the mist.

Continue to mist as needed.

Clean King

What you will need:

10 drops eucalyptus oil

10 drops grapefruit oil

Direct Application Directions:

Mix the blend well, and if you are going to apply it directly to your skin mix with 2 teaspoons sweet almond oil and spread over the affected area. You may also mix with the lotion of your choice – do not ingest the oils.

Repeat every couple hours, or as often as needed.

Diffuser Directions:

Fill your diffuser with water according to the directions on the packaging, then add a few drops of this blend, also according to the packaging. Plug in your diffuser and place it where you will be able to sit or sleep nearby, and breathe in the mist.

Continue to mist as needed.

Wellness

What you will need:

12 drops vanilla oil

10 drops cinnamon oil

Direct Application Directions:

Mix the blend well, and if you are going to apply it directly to your skin mix with 2 teaspoons sweet almond oil and spread over the affected area. You may also mix with the lotion of your choice – do not ingest the oils.

Repeat every couple hours, or as often as needed.

Diffuser Directions:

Fill your diffuser with water according to the directions on the packaging, then add a few drops of this blend, also according to the packaging. Plug in your diffuser and place it where you will be able to sit or sleep nearby, and breathe in the mist.

Continue to mist as needed.

What you will need:

12 drops orange oil

12 drops grapefruit oil

Direct Application Directions:

Mix the blend well, and if you are going to apply it directly to your skin mix with 2 teaspoons sweet almond oil and spread over the affected area. You may also mix with the lotion of your choice – do not ingest the oils.

Repeat every couple hours, or as often as needed.

Diffuser Directions:

Fill your diffuser with water according to the directions on the packaging, then add a few drops of this blend, also according to the packaging. Plug in your diffuser and place it where you will be able to sit or sleep nearby, and breathe in the mist.

Continue to mist as needed.

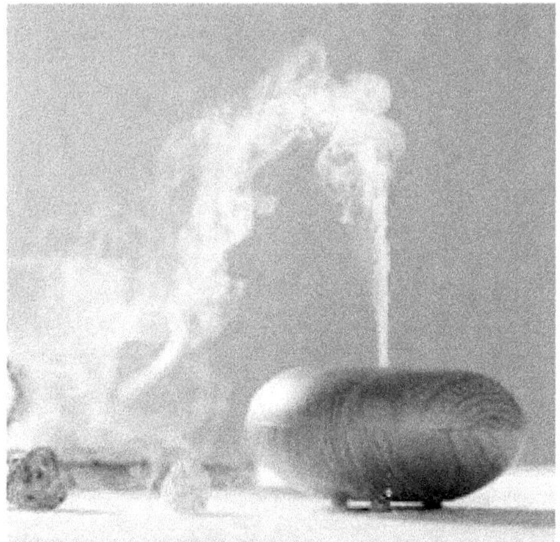

Arthritis Eraser

What you will need:

12 drops grapefruit oil

10 drops lemon oil

Direct Application Directions:

Mix the blend well, and if you are going to apply it directly to your skin mix with 2 teaspoons sweet almond oil and spread over the affected area. You may also mix with the lotion of your choice – do not ingest the oils.

Repeat every couple hours, or as often as needed.

Diffuser Directions:

Fill your diffuser with water according to the directions on the packaging, then add a few drops of this blend, also according to the packaging. Plug in your diffuser and place it where you will be able to sit or sleep nearby, and breathe in the mist.

Continue to mist as needed.

Breathe Right

What you will need:

10 drops bergamot oil

9 drops blood orange oil

Direct Application Directions:

Mix the blend well, and if you are going to apply it directly to your skin mix with 2 teaspoons sweet almond oil and spread over the affected area. You may also mix with the lotion of your choice – do not ingest the oils.

Repeat every couple hours, or as often as needed.

Diffuser Directions:

Fill your diffuser with water according to the directions on the packaging, then add a few drops of this blend, also according to the packaging. Plug in your diffuser and place it where you will be able to sit or sleep nearby, and breathe in the mist.

Continue to mist as needed.

Headache Soother

What you will need:

12 drops peppermint oil

8 drops eucalyptus oil

Direct Application Directions:

Mix the blend well, and if you are going to apply it directly to your skin mix with 2 teaspoons sweet almond oil and spread over the affected area. You may also mix with the lotion of your choice – do not ingest the oils.

Repeat every couple hours, or as often as needed.

Diffuser Directions:

Fill your diffuser with water according to the directions on the packaging, then add a few drops of this blend, also according to the packaging. Plug in your

diffuser and place it where you will be able to sit or sleep nearby, and breathe in the mist.

Continue to mist as needed.

Sleep Well
What you will need:

12 drops lavender oil

10 drops myrrh oil

Direct Application Directions:

Mix the blend well, and if you are going to apply it directly to your skin mix with 2 teaspoons sweet almond oil and spread over the affected area. You may also mix with the lotion of your choice – do not ingest the oils.

Repeat every couple hours, or as often as needed.

Diffuser Directions:

Fill your diffuser with water according to the directions on the packaging, then add a few drops of this blend, also according to the packaging. Plug in your diffuser and place it where you will be able to sit or sleep nearby, and breathe in the mist.

Continue to mist as needed.

Fever Fighter
What you will need:

10 drops vetiver oil

8 drops winter green oil

Direct Application Directions:

Mix the blend well, and if you are going to apply it directly to your skin mix with 2 teaspoons sweet almond oil and spread over the affected area. You may also mix with the lotion of your choice – do not ingest the oils.

Repeat every couple hours, or as often as needed.

Diffuser Directions:

Fill your diffuser with water according to the directions on the packaging, then add a few drops of this blend, also according to the packaging. Plug in your diffuser and place it where you will be able to sit or sleep nearby, and breathe in the mist.

Continue to mist as needed.

The Good Stuff
What you will need:

12 drops basil oil

10 drops ginger oil

Direct Application Directions:

Mix the blend well, and if you are going to apply it directly to your skin mix with 2 teaspoons sweet almond oil and spread over the affected area. You may also mix with the lotion of your choice – do not ingest the oils.

Repeat every couple hours, or as often as needed.

Diffuser Directions:

Fill your diffuser with water according to the directions on the packaging, then add a few drops of this blend, also according to the packaging. Plug in your diffuser and place it where you will be able to sit or sleep nearby, and breathe in the mist.

Continue to mist as needed.

Healthy Living
What you will need:

10 drops tea tree oil

8 drops eucalyptus oil

Direct Application Directions:

Mix the blend well, and if you are going to apply it directly to your skin mix with 2 teaspoons sweet almond oil and spread over the affected area. You may also mix with the lotion of your choice – do not ingest the oils.

Repeat every couple hours, or as often as needed.

Diffuser Directions:

Fill your diffuser with water according to the directions on the packaging, then add a few drops of this blend, also according to the packaging. Plug in your diffuser and place it where you will be able to sit or sleep nearby, and breathe in the mist.

Continue to mist as needed.

I Can Breathe
What you will need:

12 drops peppermint

10 drops eucalyptus

Direct Application Directions:

Mix the blend well, and if you are going to apply it directly to your skin mix with 2 teaspoons sweet almond oil and spread over the affected area. You may also mix with the lotion of your choice – do not ingest the oils.

Repeat every couple hours, or as often as needed.

Diffuser Directions:

Fill your diffuser with water according to the directions on the packaging, then add a few drops of this blend, also according to the packaging. Plug in your diffuser and place it where you will be able to sit or sleep nearby, and breathe in the mist.

Continue to mist as needed.

Cough Stopper

What you will need:

10 drops frankincense

12 drops peppermint oil

Direct Application Directions:

Mix the blend well, and if you are going to apply it directly to your skin mix with 2 teaspoons sweet almond oil and spread over the affected area. You may also mix with the lotion of your choice – do not ingest the oils.

Repeat every couple hours, or as often as needed.

Diffuser Directions:

Fill your diffuser with water according to the directions on the packaging, then add a few drops of this blend, also according to the packaging. Plug in your diffuser and place it where you will be able to sit or sleep nearby, and breathe in the mist.

Continue to mist as needed.

Better Than Meds
What you will need:

10 drops lemon oil

12 drops rose oil

Direct Application Directions:

Mix the blend well, and if you are going to apply it directly to your skin mix with 2 teaspoons sweet almond oil and spread over the affected area. You may also mix with the lotion of your choice – do not ingest the oils.

Repeat every couple hours, or as often as needed.

Diffuser Directions:

Fill your diffuser with water according to the directions on the packaging, then add a few drops of this blend, also according to the packaging. Plug in your diffuser and place it where you will be able to sit or sleep nearby, and breathe in the mist.

Continue to mist as needed.

Germaphobe

What you will need:

10 drops peppermint oil

10 drops lemon oil

Direct Application Directions:

Mix the blend well, and if you are going to apply it directly to your skin mix with 2 teaspoons sweet almond oil and spread over the affected area. You may also mix with the lotion of your choice – do not ingest the oils.

Repeat every couple hours, or as often as needed.

Diffuser Directions:

Fill your diffuser with water according to the directions on the packaging, then add a few drops of this blend, also according to the packaging. Plug in your diffuser and place it where you will be able to sit or sleep nearby, and breathe in the mist.

Continue to mist as needed.

Hercules

What you will need:

12 drops bergamot oil

10 drops rosemary oil

Direct Application Directions:

Mix the blend well, and if you are going to apply it directly to your skin mix with 2 teaspoons sweet almond oil and spread over the affected area. You may also mix with the lotion of your choice – do not ingest the oils.

Repeat every couple hours, or as often as needed.

Diffuser Directions:

Fill your diffuser with water according to the directions on the packaging, then add a few drops of this blend, also according to the packaging. Plug in your diffuser and place it where you will be able to sit or sleep nearby, and breathe in the mist.

Continue to mist as needed.

Bacteria Be Gone
What you will need:

8 drops blood orange oil

5 drops tea tree oil

Direct Application Directions:

Mix the blend well, and if you are going to apply it directly to your skin mix with 2 teaspoons sweet almond oil and spread over the affected area. You may also mix with the lotion of your choice – do not ingest the oils.

Repeat every couple hours, or as often as needed.

Diffuser Directions:

Fill your diffuser with water according to the directions on the packaging, then add a few drops of this blend, also according to the packaging. Plug in your diffuser and place it where you will be able to sit or sleep nearby, and breathe in the mist.

Continue to mist as needed.

Germ's Worst Nightmare

What you will need:

12 drops orange oil

10 drops lemon oil

Direct Application Directions:

Mix the blend well, and if you are going to apply it directly to your skin mix with 2 teaspoons sweet almond oil and spread over the affected area. You may also mix with the lotion of your choice – do not ingest the oils.

Repeat every couple hours, or as often as needed.

Diffuser Directions:

Fill your diffuser with water according to the directions on the packaging, then add a few drops of this blend, also according to the packaging. Plug in your diffuser and place it where you will be able to sit or sleep nearby, and breathe in the mist.

Continue to mist as needed.

The Ancient Way

What you will need:

10 drops chamomile

9 drops clary sage oil

Direct Application Directions:

Mix the blend well, and if you are going to apply it directly to your skin mix with 2 teaspoons sweet almond oil and spread over the affected area. You may also mix with the lotion of your choice – do not ingest the oils.

Repeat every couple hours, or as often as needed.

Diffuser Directions:

Fill your diffuser with water according to the directions on the packaging, then add a few drops of this blend, also according to the packaging. Plug in your diffuser and place it where you will be able to sit or sleep nearby, and breathe in the mist.

Continue to mist as needed.

Best Blend
What you will need:

8 drops frankincense oil

11 drops goldenseal oil

Direct Application Directions:

Mix the blend well, and if you are going to apply it directly to your skin mix with 2 teaspoons sweet almond oil and spread over the affected area. You may also mix with the lotion of your choice – do not ingest the oils.

Repeat every couple hours, or as often as needed.

Diffuser Directions:

Fill your diffuser with water according to the directions on the packaging, then add a few drops of this blend, also according to the packaging. Plug in your diffuser and place it where you will be able to sit or sleep nearby, and breathe in the mist.

Continue to mist as needed.

Health Tonic

What you will need:

10 drops geranium oil

10 drops rose oil

Direct Application Directions:

Mix the blend well, and if you are going to apply it directly to your skin mix with 2 teaspoons sweet almond oil and spread over the affected area. You may also mix with the lotion of your choice – do not ingest the oils.

Repeat every couple hours, or as often as needed.

Diffuser Directions:

Fill your diffuser with water according to the directions on the packaging, then add a few drops of this blend, also according to the packaging. Plug in your diffuser and place it where you will be able to sit or sleep nearby, and breathe in the mist.

Continue to mist as needed.

Toxin Basher

What you will need:

12 drops clary sage oil

8 drops sage oil

Direct Application Directions:

Mix the blend well, and if you are going to apply it directly to your skin mix with 2 teaspoons sweet almond oil and spread over the affected area. You may also mix with the lotion of your choice – do not ingest the oils.

Repeat every couple hours, or as often as needed.

Diffuser Directions:

Fill your diffuser with water according to the directions on the packaging, then add a few drops of this blend, also according to the packaging. Plug in your diffuser and place it where you will be able to sit or sleep nearby, and breathe in the mist.

Continue to mist as needed.

Sick Days

What you will need:

12 drops vetiver oil

10 drops cardamom oil

Direct Application Directions:

Mix the blend well, and if you are going to apply it directly to your skin mix with 2 teaspoons sweet almond oil and spread over the affected area. You may also mix with the lotion of your choice – do not ingest the oils.

Repeat every couple hours, or as often as needed.

Diffuser Directions:

Fill your diffuser with water according to the directions on the packaging, then add a few drops of this blend, also according to the packaging. Plug in your diffuser and place it where you will be able to sit or sleep nearby, and breathe in the mist.

Continue to mist as needed.

Flu Diffuser

What you will need:

10 drops tea tree oil

12 drops sandalwood oil

Direct Application Directions:

Mix the blend well, and if you are going to apply it directly to your skin mix with 2 teaspoons sweet almond oil and spread over the affected area. You may also mix with the lotion of your choice – do not ingest the oils.

Repeat every couple hours, or as often as needed.

Diffuser Directions:

Fill your diffuser with water according to the directions on the packaging, then add a few drops of this blend, also according to the packaging. Plug in your diffuser and place it where you will be able to sit or sleep nearby, and breathe in the mist.

Continue to mist as needed.

Tummy Ache Soother

What you will need:

12 drops peppermint oil

10 drops spearmint oil

Direct Application Directions:

Mix the blend well, and if you are going to apply it directly to your skin mix with 2 teaspoons sweet almond oil and spread over the affected area. You may also mix with the lotion of your choice – do not ingest the oils.

Repeat every couple hours, or as often as needed.

Diffuser Directions:

Fill your diffuser with water according to the directions on the packaging, then add a few drops of this blend, also according to the packaging. Plug in your diffuser and place it where you will be able to sit or sleep nearby, and breathe in the mist.

Continue to mist as needed.

Just What the Doctor Ordered
What you will need:

10 drops chamomile oil

8 drops ylang ylang

Direct Application Directions:

Mix the blend well, and if you are going to apply it directly to your skin mix with 2 teaspoons sweet almond oil and spread over the affected area. You may also mix with the lotion of your choice – do not ingest the oils.

Repeat every couple hours, or as often as needed.

Diffuser Directions:

Fill your diffuser with water according to the directions on the packaging, then add a few drops of this blend, also according to the packaging. Plug in your diffuser and place it where you will be able to sit or sleep nearby, and breathe in the mist.

Continue to mist as needed.

Mom's Blend

What you will need:

10 drops geranium oil

7 drops ginger oil

Direct Application Directions:

Mix the blend well, and if you are going to apply it directly to your skin mix with 2 teaspoons sweet almond oil and spread over the affected area. You may also mix with the lotion of your choice – do not ingest the oils.

Repeat every couple hours, or as often as needed.

Diffuser Directions:

Fill your diffuser with water according to the directions on the packaging, then add a few drops of this blend, also according to the packaging. Plug in your diffuser and place it where you will be able to sit or sleep nearby, and breathe in the mist.

Continue to mist as needed.

It's in the Air

What you will need:

8 drops frankincense

5 drops tea tree oil

Direct Application Directions:

Mix the blend well, and if you are going to apply it directly to your skin mix with 2 teaspoons sweet almond oil and spread over the affected area. You may also mix with the lotion of your choice – do not ingest the oils.

Repeat every couple hours, or as often as needed.

Diffuser Directions:

Fill your diffuser with water according to the directions on the packaging, then add a few drops of this blend, also according to the packaging. Plug in your diffuser and place it where you will be able to sit or sleep nearby, and breathe in the mist.

Continue to mist as needed.

Conclusion

There you have it, everything you need to create blends to heal any illness and keep your family healthy and strong. When you take care of your health the natural way, you get all the great benefits that come with healthy living, and none of the harmful side effects that come with medication.

With this book, you can step out of the conventional way of doing things and into a lifestyle that is both natural and healthy. Do the right thing for yourself and your family, and step into the world of healthy living.

Good luck and stay healthy.